**Yoshiro Fujii**

# Electromagnetic waves and indirect effect

Yoshiro Fujii

# Electromagnetic waves and indirect effect

**Don't you believe anything which isn't visible?**

**LAP LAMBERT Academic Publishing**

**Imprint**

Any brand names and product names mentioned in this book are subject to trademark, brand or patent protection and are trademarks or registered trademarks of their respective holders. The use of brand names, product names, common names, trade names, product descriptions etc. even without a particular marking in this work is in no way to be construed to mean that such names may be regarded as unrestricted in respect of trademark and brand protection legislation and could thus be used by anyone.

Cover image: www.ingimage.com

Publisher:
LAP LAMBERT Academic Publishing
is a trademark of
Dodo Books Indian Ocean Ltd. and OmniScriptum S.R.L publishing group

120 High Road, East Finchley, London, N2 9ED, United Kingdom
Str. Armeneasca 28/1, office 1, Chisinau MD-2012, Republic of Moldova, Europe
Managing Directors: Ieva Konstantinova, Victoria Ursu
info@omniscriptum.com

Printed at: see last page
**ISBN: 978-3-659-69995-5**

Copyright © Yoshiro Fujii
Copyright © 2015 Dodo Books Indian Ocean Ltd. and OmniScriptum S.R.L publishing group

# Electromagnetic waves and indirect effect

Don't you believe anything which isn't visible?

Yoshiro Fujii, DDS. Ph.D.

|        | Table of contents | Pages |
|--------|-------------------|-------|
| Case 1 | Treatment of sever lumbago | 3 |
|        | Subject and Methods | 3 |
|        | Results | 5 |
|        | In terms of Bi-Digital O-Ring Test | 7 |
|        | Discussion | 8 |
| Case 2 | In direct and direct effect of a denture | 8 |
|        | Subject, Methods, and Results | 8 |
| Case 3 | Hip joint pain after a surgical operation on the humerus | 11 |
|        | Subject, Methods, and Results | 11 |
|        | Discussion | 13 |
| Case 4 | The electromagnetic waves emitted by a cell phone forced a subject to lean. | 14 |
| Case 5 | Hip joint pain after a surgical operation on the humerus | 16 |
|        | Subject, Methods, and Results | 16 |
|        | Discussion | 23 |
| Case 6 | Instability of jaw position | 24 |
|        | Subject, Methods, and Results | 24 |
|        | Discussion | 28 |
| Case 7 | Difficulty of head movement | 30 |
|        | Subject, Methods, and Results | 30 |
|        | Discussion | 32 |
| Case 8 | Effect of magnetic field on the body | 33 |
|        | Subject and Methods | 33 |
|        | Results | 34 |
|        | Discussion | 36 |

| **Case 9** | Indirect and direct effect of a small denture on the whole body | 36 |
| **Case 10** | Lumbago due a lumber vertebra herniated disc was treated by the indirect effect of medicine | 42 |
| | Subject, Methods, and Results | 42 |
| | Discussion | 45 |

Overall discussion     45

Conclusion     49

# Electromagnetic waves and indirect effect

Don't you believe anything which isn't visible?

Yoshiro Fujii, DDS. Ph.D.

I started this research because of the incident described below. One day, a patient came my dental clinic to cure her knee pain because there is a close relationship between the biting conditions and knee conditions [1]. I thought that her knee trouble was related to her biting condition. Therefore, I asked her to remove her denture. While her denture was removed, I adjusted it near her. While I was adjusting it, the patient reported that her knee pain had disappeared. I was very surprised because her denture was not placed in her mouth. Next, I moved her denture away from her. The pain in her knee recurred. I did not understand why such a result occurred. However, I have seen similar results time after time in my clinical work. When a substance was brought close to a subject, the effect of that substance on the subject's body increased. When the substance was moved away from the subject, the effect decreased. When the subject was shield from the substance with aluminum foil, the effect of the substance also decreased. As a result, I imagined that something like electromagnetic waves was being emitted by the substances and that these 'waves' were influencing the physical condition of my patients. I would like to give you some more detailed examples.

.

## Case 1: Treatment of sever lumbago

Subject and Methods

The subject was a woman in her 40s. She had suffered from lumbago for a long time. The subject underwent a variety of non-surgical treatments. However, none were found to be effective; therefore, the doctor-in-charge recommended that she visit my dental clinic for treatment. She could barely bend forward at the waist because of her lumbago (Figure 1). So, I set a gold alloy metal crown (Au 87%, Pt 10.6% and the other) which was judged to be effective by the Bi-Digital O-Ring Test [2, 3], on her upper first molar (Figure 2).

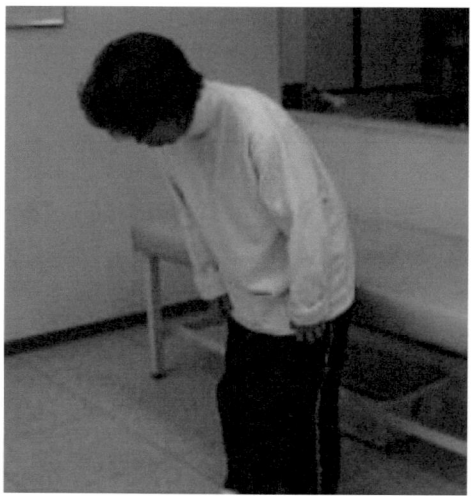

Figure 1: The subject suffered from lumbago for a long time and could not bend forward because of the back pain.

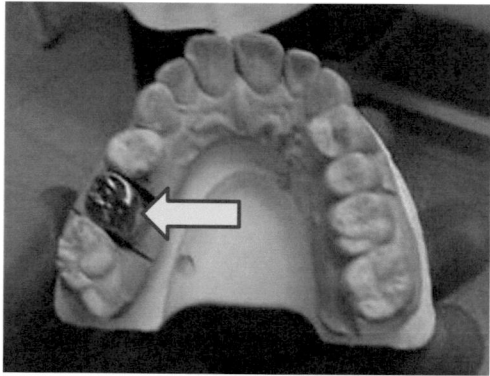

Figure 2: A gold alloy metal crown was set on her right upper first molar (arrow).

Results

As soon as the gold alloy metal crown was placed on the floor just in front of her feet, she was able to touch the floor very easily and her lumbago markedly improved (Figure 3). When the crown was covered with aluminum foil, the symptoms recurred, and it became very difficult for her to bend her body forward (Figure 4); however, when the aluminum foil was removed, she could easily bend forward again. After the crown was set in her mouth (Figure 5), the state of her lower back improved more than that shown in Figure 3 (Figure 6). I followed the subject's condition for about five years after her crown was placed. During that time her lumbago did not recur and she did not use any other treatments because she was satisfied with her condition.

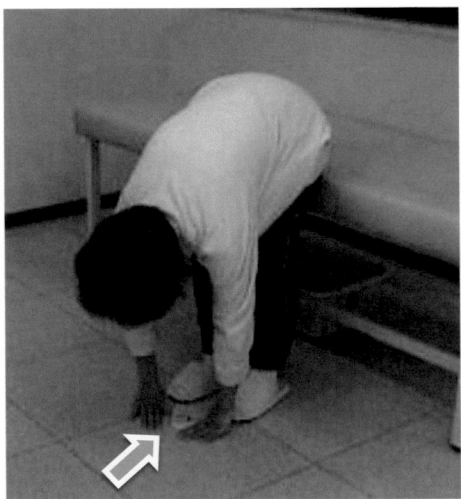

Figure 3: As soon as the gold alloy metal crown (arrow) was placed on the floor just in front of her feet, she was able to touch the floor very easily and her lumbago markedly improved

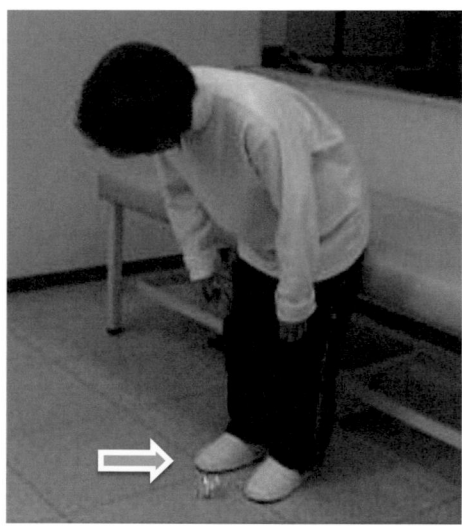

Figure 4: She could barely bend forward after the crown was covered with aluminum foil (arrow).

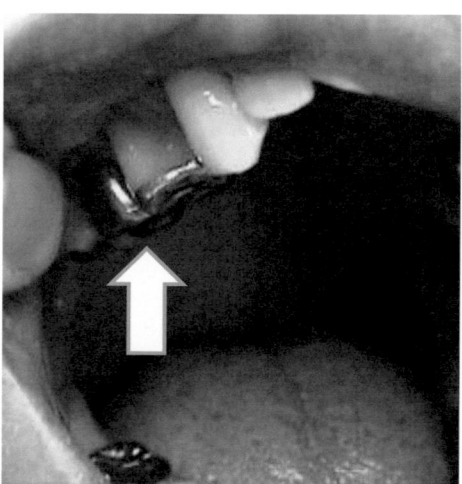

Figure 5: The crown was set in the subject's mouth (arrow)

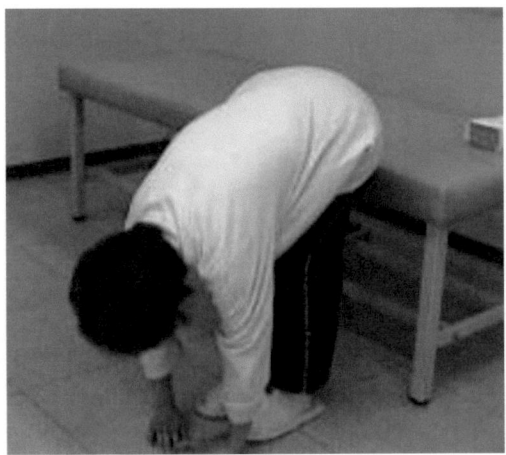

Figure 6: After the crown was set in her mouth, she was able to bend forward even farther than she was when the crown was on the floor in front of her (Figure 3)

In order to watch the actual experiment described in this case, please visit the YouTube movie:
Lumbago improves by simply placing a crown near foot
https://www.youtube.com/watch?v=FoTSWuVw24s&list=UUqAoDvLMJAJ-H-HLCF4V8-A
(last checked: 8 Jan 2015)

In terms of the Bi-Digital O-Ring Test

The Bi-Digital O-Ring Test [2,3] is a subjective evaluation of a patient's opposing muscle strength in which a diagnostician employs the thumb and forefinger of each hand, formed in the shape of an O, to attempt to force apart an O shape formed by the patient who places the fingertips of their thumb and one of their remaining fingers together. At the same time, the patient holds a slide of organ tissue, a sample of medication, potential allergen, etc., in their free hand. The diagnostician then uses their perception of the strength required to force apart the patient's 'O-ring' of thumb and one of the remaining fingers to assess the patient's health [2,3]. It is very useful to judge the effect of the object (i.e. dental materials).

Discussion

Although the crown was placed near the subject's foot, not in her mouth, her lumbago improved immediately. This phenomenon can be interfered from the results of covering the crown with aluminum foil. I believe that something like electromagnetic waves had an effect on her lumbago. The generally accepted theory is that if a substance is not in the body, it will have no effect. However, I have noticed that even when substances are not in the body, they can have a marked effect. In some cases, just bringing the substance close to the body can have an effect. This study revealed that even when substances do not enter the body, they can have a marked effect on joint mobility. This appears to be true even when the substances are simply in close proximity to the body, indicating that a substance can influence a patient's condition in three ways: 1) the substance can be placed or absorbed by the cells, 2) it can have an effect when in close proximity to the body, and 3) it can cause a placebo effect. The author suggests that the first mechanism be called the "direct effect" of the substance and the second be called "the indirect effect". Therefore, the outcome of setting the crown in her mouth was the sum of the direct and indirect effects of the crown on the patient. The direct effect included restoration of occlusion, restoration of tooth contact, positioning of buccal part and tongue, and other esthetic changes. The indirect effect was like electromagnetic waves emitted by the crown.

## Case 2: In direct and direct effect of a denture

Subject, Methods, and Results

The subject was a woman in her 60s. Before this experiment, she was blindfolded (Figure 7). She had a lower full denture which was made by the author (Figure 8). It was judged to be effective by the Bi-Digital O-Ring Test [2, 3].

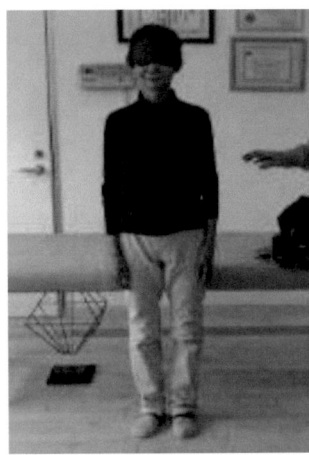

Figure 7: The subject was blindfolded before this experiment.

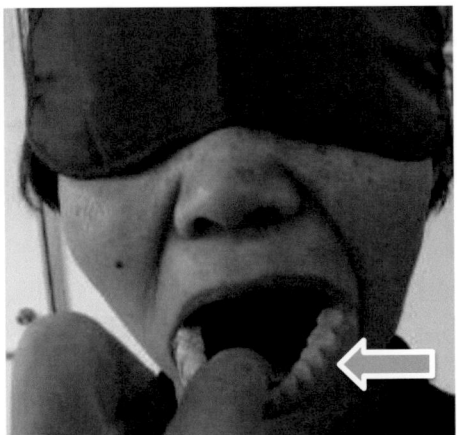

Figure 8: She had a lower full denture (arrow).

It was made of resin (Polymethyl methacrylate) and alloy (Au 87%, Pt 11% the other). When she bent forward while blindfolded without her denture, the distance between her finger tips and the floor (FFD) was about 3cm (Figure 9). When the denture was secretly placed near her feet, she was able to touch the floor with her fingertips (Figure 10).

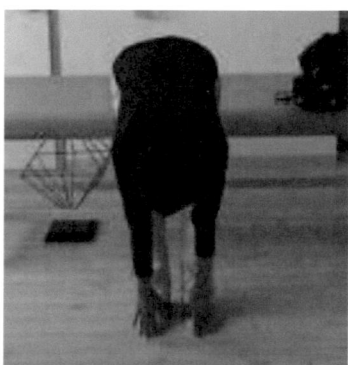

Figure 9: When she bent forward while blindfolded without her denture, she could not touch the floor. Her FFD (Distance between fingertips and floor) was about 3cm.

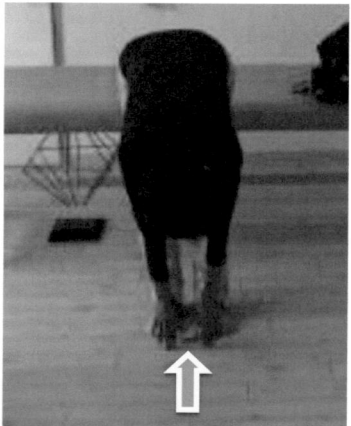

Figure 10: When the denture (arrow) was secretly placed near her feet, she was able to touch the floor with her fingertips.

When the denture was removed, she was unable to keep her fingertips on the floor because of the tension of her legs. When the denture was placed in her mouth, she could bend more easily than when the denture was placed near her feet (Figure 11).

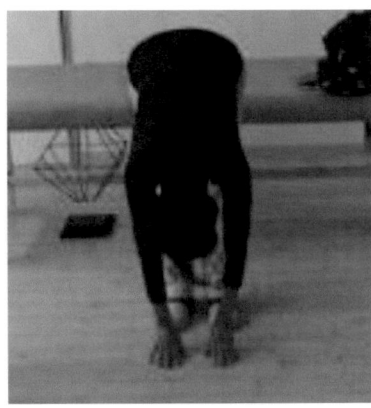

Figure 11: When the denture was placed in her mouth, she could bend more easily than when the denture was placed near her feet

In order to watch the actual experiment described in this case, please visit the YouTube movie:
Lumbago improves by simply placing a crown near foot
https://www.youtube.com/watch?v=JcW9MQG_-Ww
(last checked: 8 Jan 2015)

## Case 3: Hip joint pain after a surgical operation on the humerus

Subject, Methods, and Results

The subject was a woman in her 20s. She sustained a compound fracture of her left humerus in an accident (Figure 12). She needed to have an operation to repair the bone. Seven titanium screws were inserted (Figure 13).

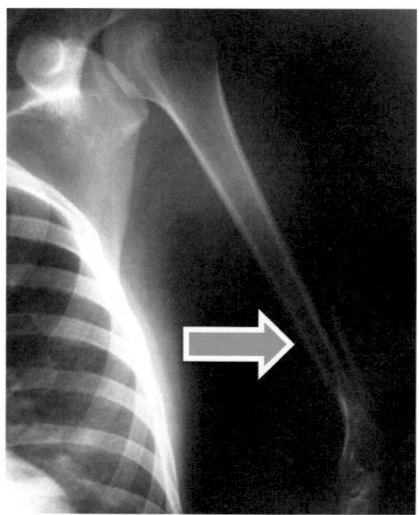

Figure12: Her left humerus had a compound fracture (arrow).

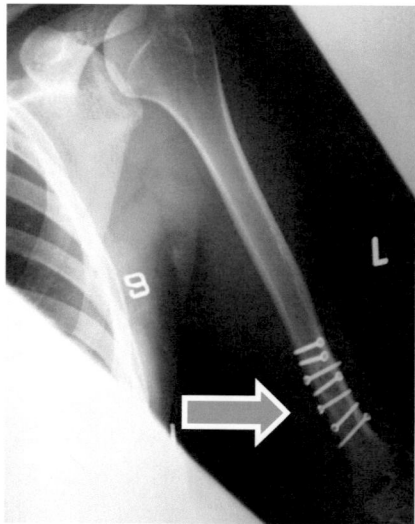

Figure 13: seven titanium screws were surgically implanted (arrow).

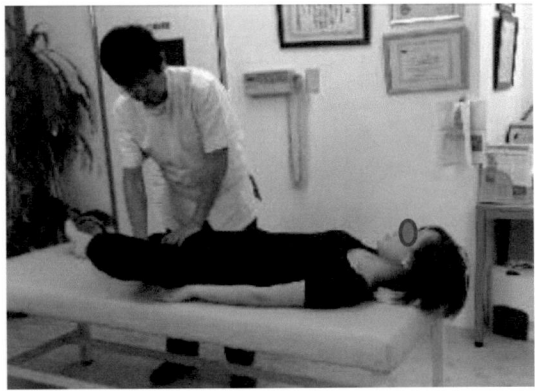

Figure 14: When outwardly rotating her left hip joint, she could not lower her left knee completely due to pain and tension.

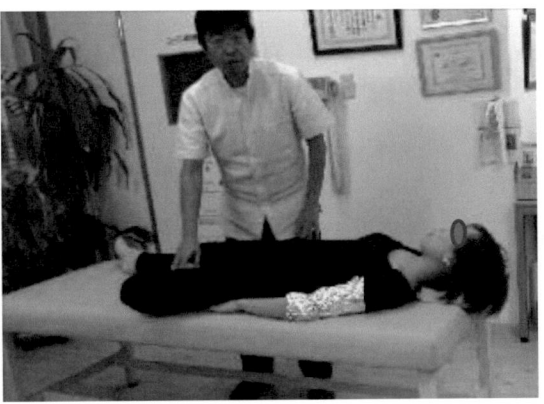

Figure 15: When her left upper arm was covered with aluminum foil, she was able to lower left knee to the table top.

Discussion

The titanium screws implanted in the subject's humerus might be collecting harmful electromagnetic waves. I have previously reported that harmful electromagnetic waves may induce joint mobility disorder [4]. In such a case, removing the screws is recommended, however, the surgical doctor in-charge did not agree with removal because he did not understand this theory. Following the tests described above, and my diagnosis, the subject began to wrap in aluminum foil around her upper left arm regularly in order to suppress her joint pain.

In order to watch the actual experiment described in this case, please visit the YouTube movie:
Hip joint pain caused by surgical screws implanted in the upper arm.
https://www.youtube.com/watch?v=dqZIizMDQ70
(last checked: 2 Apr 2015)

## Case 4: The electromagnetic waves emitted by a cell phone forced a subject to lean.

I have observed that some subjects usually involuntarily lean away from (rarely approach to) an active cell phone because of the electromagnetic waves being emitted (Figure 16).

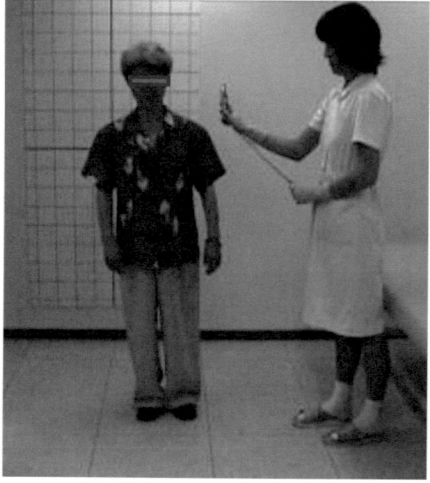

Figure 16: The subject was forced to lean away by the electromagnetic waves being emitted by the cell phone.

The reason why such a phenomenon occurs is still unclear. However, it is confirmed that electromagnetic waves emitted by cell phones may induce balance dysregulation. Dental materials sometimes act as antennas which collect electromagnetic waves. When the electromagnetic waves collected by dental materials are harmful to the body, unpleasant symptoms (electromagnetic hypersensitivity) may occur. With development of an Information Technology (IT) society, the opportunity to use electronic devices, such as cell phones and personal computers, has become increasingly widespread and has enabled communication on a global scale [5, 6]. However, there have been many reports pertaining to health problems resulting from the electromagnetic waves emitted by such electronic devices [7-14]. Physically unpleasant symptoms including headache, fatigue, tinnitus, dizziness, memory loss, irregular heartbeat, and whole-body skin lesions caused by exposure to electromagnetic waves, are recognized as electromagnetic hypersensitivity (EHS) [15-19]. I have reported that scoliosis can develop from exposure to electromagnetic waves [20]. I have also reported how a subject's involuntary movements, caused by electromagnetic waves, were treated using a gold alloy dental inlay [21]. Additionally, I have reported how a subject's dizziness and joint mobility disorder, caused by electromagnetic waves, were treated using dental techniques [4].

Dental materials and electromagnetic waves, can interact and influence a person's condition in three important ways: First, the dental materials can collect electromagnetic waves [4, 20]. Second, they can neutralize the effects of electromagnetic waves [20]. Third, the materials can emit electromagnetic (or similar) waves (Case 1). The third point may help to explain how medicine can influence a person's condition [22]. The third point is the foundation of the indirect effect. In short, every substance emits waves, so every substance can influence a person's body functions whether it is absorbed, set in the body, or just in close proximity. This theory is not yet accepted by mainstream medicine. Such effects are often unnoticed, ignored or explained away as being the result of a placebo effect [22].

# Case 5: Hip joint and back pain after implantation of dental implants

Subject, Methods, and Results

The subject was a woman in her 50's. She developed pain in her back, hip joints, and legs about three months after the implantation of titanium dental implants in the space left by the removal of her upper right molars. There were two titanium dental implants, but there were no over-structures yet (Figure 17, 18), because of her serious body conditions.

When an active cell phone was brought close to her while she was standing, her body leaned. Her left SLR (Straight Leg Raising) and the outer rotation of her left hip joint were limited due to pain and tension (Figure 19, 20). When the implants were covered with aluminum foil (Figure 21), her left SLR and hip joint rotation improved (Figure 22, 23).

Therefore, the implants were removed by an oral surgeon (Figure 24). After removing the implants, her left SLR and her hip joint rotation improved (Figure 25, 26). All of her back and leg symptoms also improved. However, when the removed implants (Figure 27) were placed on her chest (Figure 28), her left SLR and hip joint rotation decreased again (Figure 29). As soon as the implants removed from her chest, her outer hip rotation increased, moreover, when an active cell phone was brought close to her while she was standing, her body no longer leaned.

The author replaced the implants with a partial denture containing gold and platinum alloy.

After this treatment her body conditions became very well. The symptoms which she had been suffering would not recur.

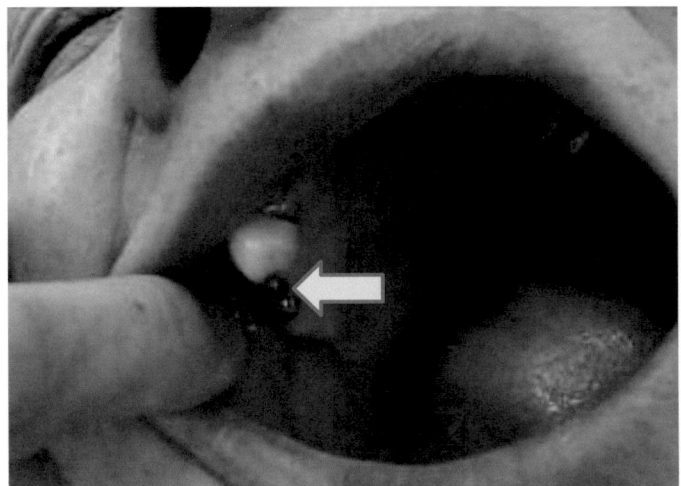

Figure 17: There were two titanium dental implants in the space left by the extraction of her upper right molars (arrow).

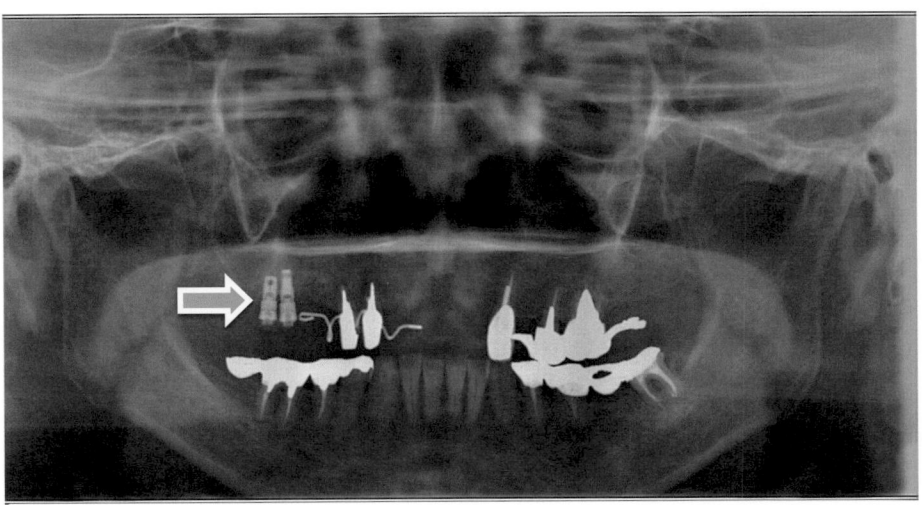

Figure 18: An panoramic X-ray image of the two titanium dental implants where her upper right molars had been (arrow).

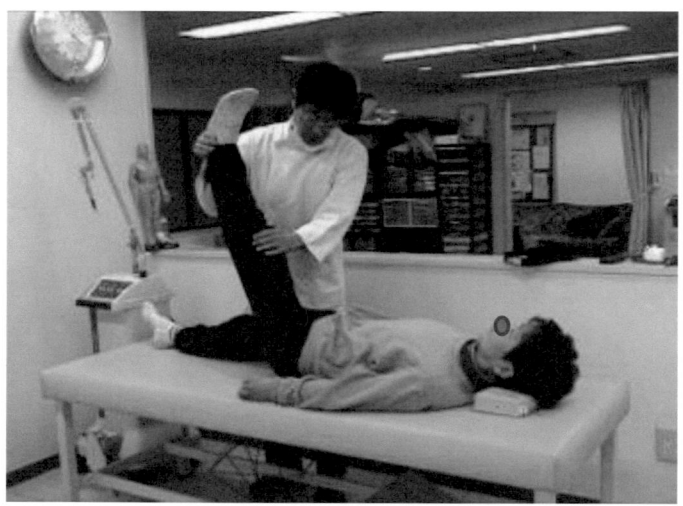

Figure 19: Her left SLR (Straight Leg Raising) was limited due to pain and tension.

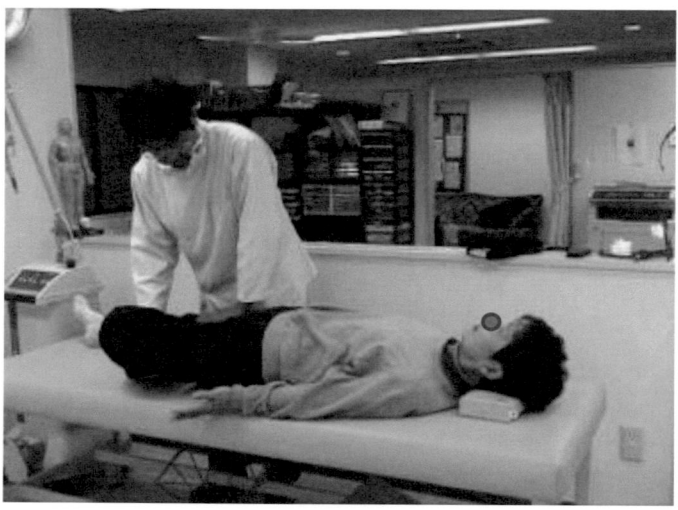

Figure 20: Her left hip joint outer rotation was limited due to pain and tension.

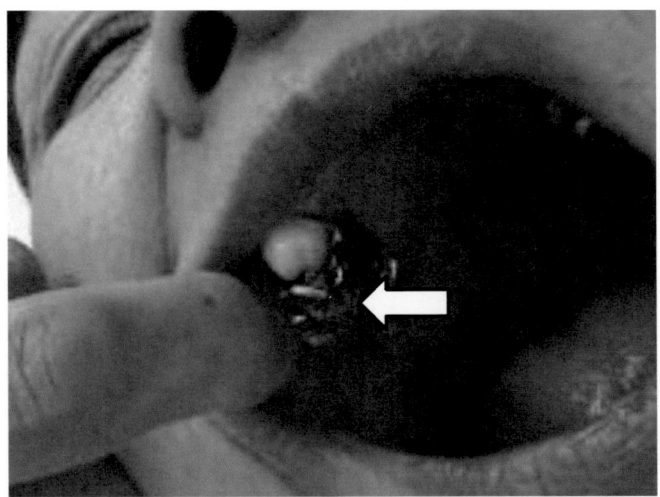

Figure 21: The implants were covered with aluminum foil (arrow).

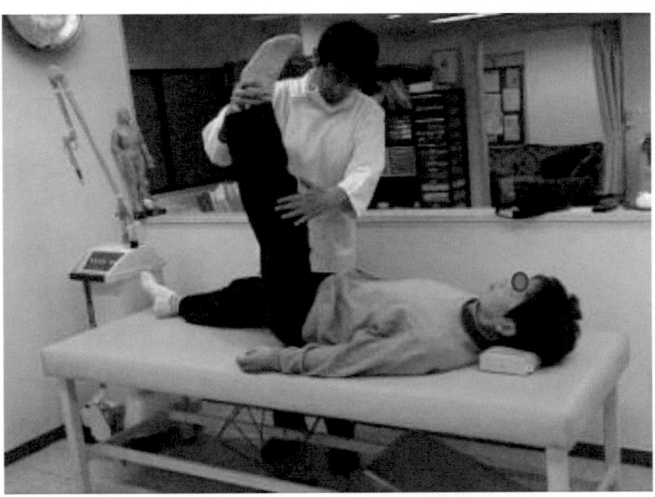

Figure 22: When the implants were covered with aluminum foil, her left SLR improved.

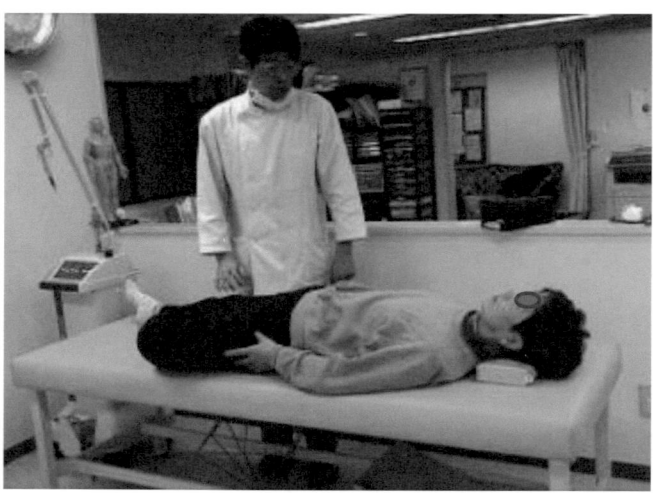

Figure 23: When the implants were covered with aluminum foil, her left hip joint outer rotation also improved.

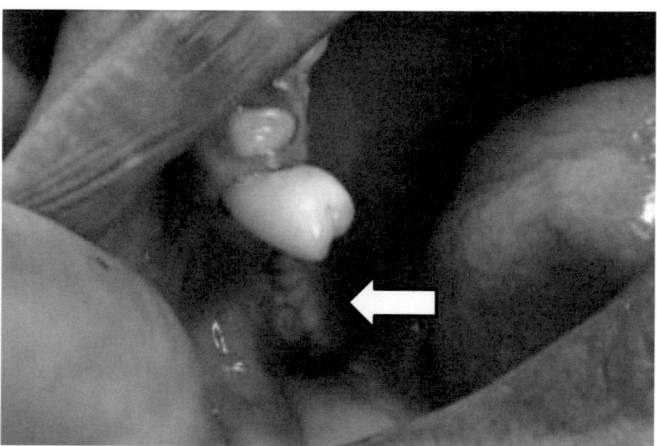

Figure 24: The implants were removed from the subject's right upper jaw. Please compare with Figure 17 (arrow).

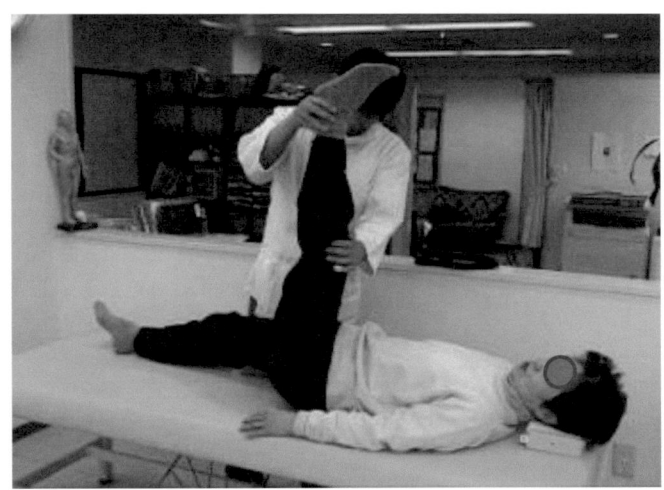

Figure 25: After the removal of implants, her left SLR improved.

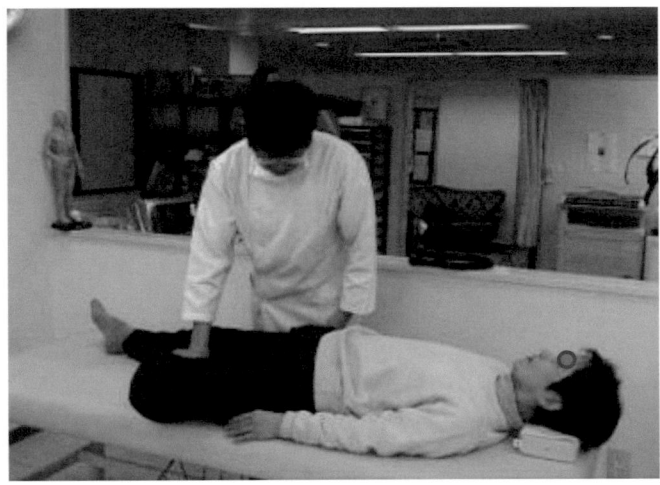

Figure 26: After the removal of the implants, her left hip joint rotation also improved.

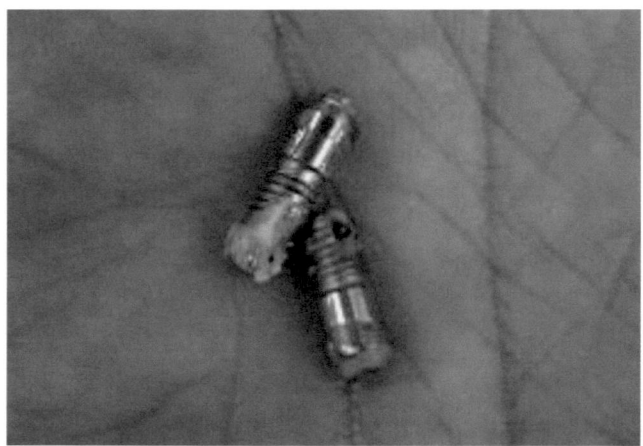

Figure 27: The two titanium implants which were removed.

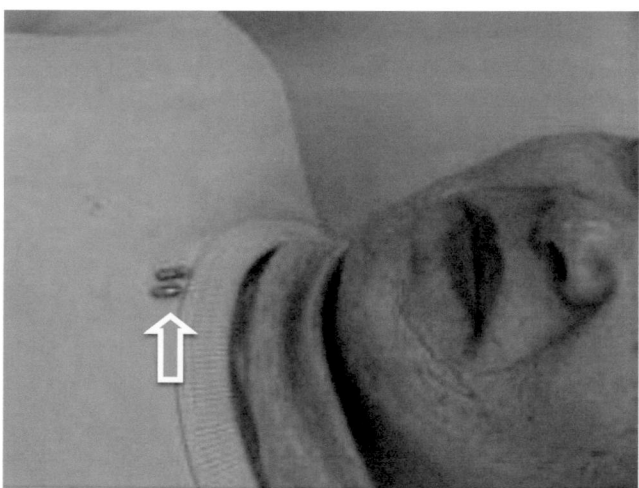

Figure 28: The two removed implants were placed on her chest (arrow).

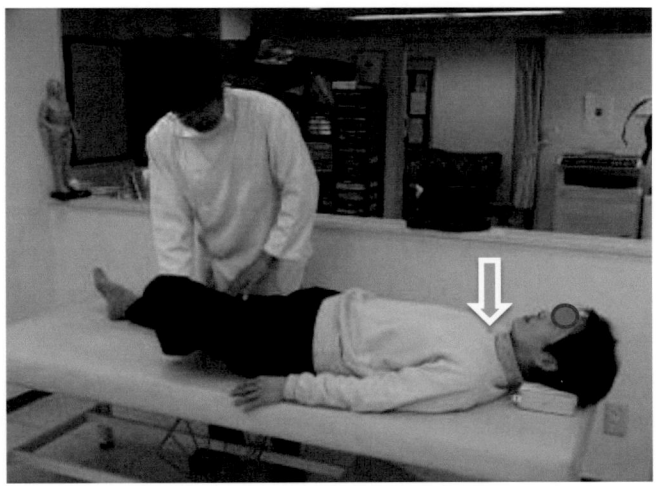

Figure 29: When the implants were placed on her chest (arrow), her left SLR and hip joint outer rotation decreased. As soon as the implants were removed, her joint movement returned.

Discussion

I have previously reported a case in which joint mobility disorder was induced by harmful electromagnetic waves [4]. I have also reported a case in which dental implants may collect harmful electromagnetic waves [20, 23]. In the current case, two titanium implants might have collected harmful electromagnetic waves and induced joint mobility disorders. Aluminum foil might have played a role in interfering with the electromagnetic waves being absorbed by the implants. Following the surgery, I made a partial denture to restore her biting condition. Her symptoms did not recur after the denture was set. Her symptoms recurred when the removed implants were placed on her chest. However, an aluminum foil covering is not a practical solution. It was not possible to cover the implants with aluminum foil. Therefore, the best option for treating the root cause of the problem was to surgically remove the implants. I told her not to keep any substances which collect harmful electromagnetic waves on or near her body after completion the dental treatment.

## Case 6: Instability of jaw position

Subject, Methods, and Results

The subject was a woman in her 60's. Her chief complaint was instability of her jaw position. Due to the instability, it was very difficult for the dentist in-charge to determine her precise biting position. Hence, her dental treatment had not succeeded. Both sides of her lower premolars and molars had temporary crowns. Her incisors and cuspids were intact (Figure 30).

When an active cell phone was brought to near her face, her jaw moved involuntarily (Figure 31). I determined that the crown which had set her right upper second molar was suspicious by using the Bi-Digital O-Ring Test (Figure 32). Then, I covered her upper right second molar cast crown with aluminum foil (Figure 33). As a result, the involuntary movement disappeared even when the active cell phone was brought close to her face (Figure 34). Therefore, I removed the crown (Figure 35, 36). After removal of the crown, her involuntary movement disappeared. In order to confirm the cause, I placed the removed crown on her cheek and bring close the active cell phone to her face, the involuntary movement of the subject recurred.

Therefore, the author replaced the cast crown with an adequate crown which was recognized good for her body by Bi-Digital O-Ring Test [2, 3]. Since her involuntary movement was disappeared and her jaw became stable, her dental treatment progressed smoothly. All temporary crowns were replaced with the appropriate materials for her body.

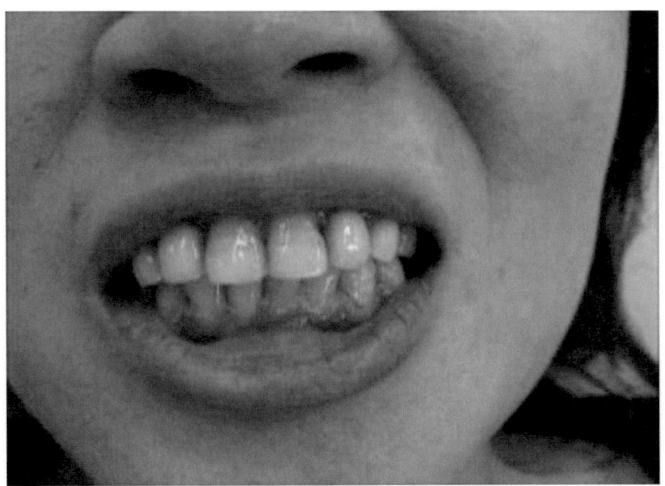

Figure 30: Before treatment. Both sides of her lower premolars and molars had temporary crowns, although her incisors and cuspids were intact.

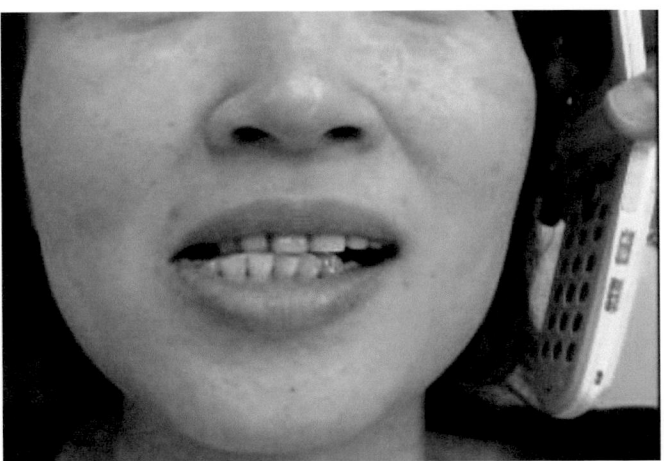

Figure 31: When an active cell phone was brought close to her cheek, her jaw moved involuntarily.

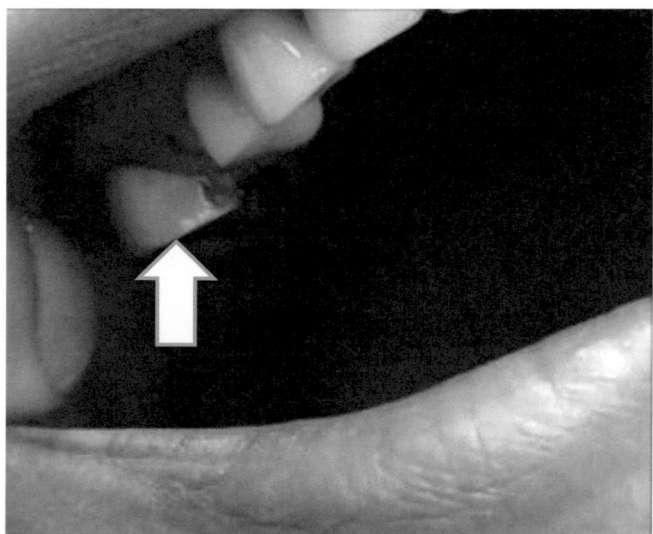

Figure 32: There is a full cast metal crown with a ceramic cover in her upper right second molar (arrow). It was judged to be suspicious using the Bi-Digital O-Ring Test.

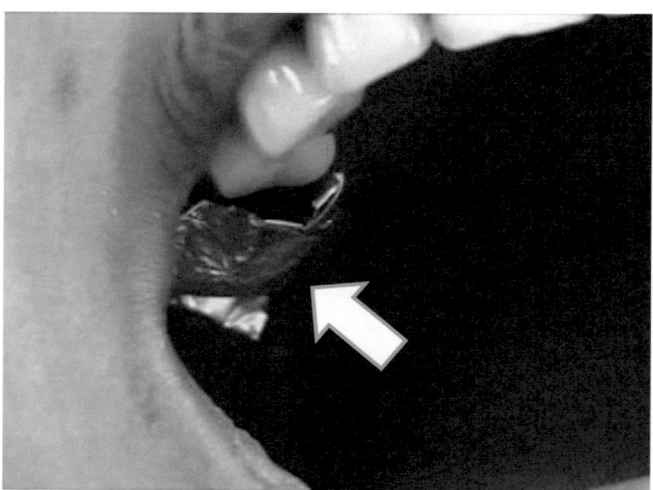

Figure 33: Her upper right second molar cast crown was covered with aluminum foil (arrow).

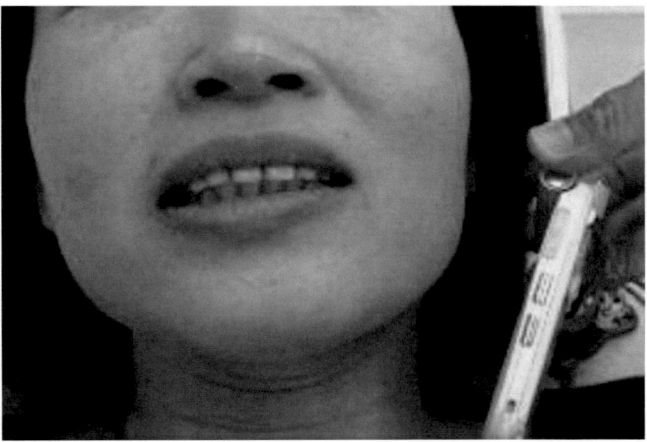

Figure 34: When her upper right second molar cast crown was covered with aluminum foil, the involuntary movement disappeared, even when the active cell phone was brought close to her cheek.

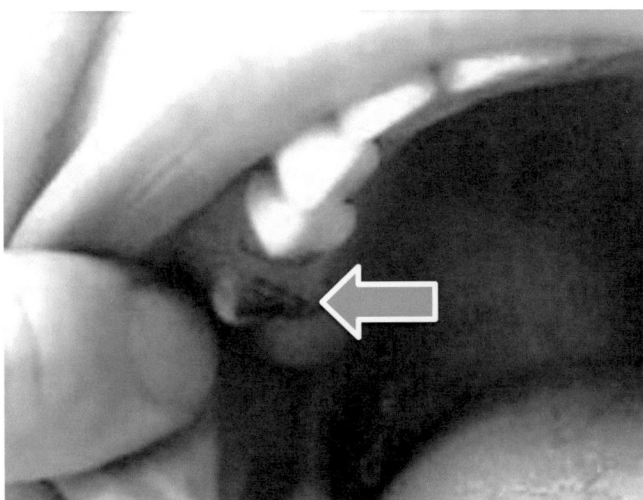

Figure 35: The crown set on her upper right second molar was removed. The arrow indicates the second molar after the crown was removed .

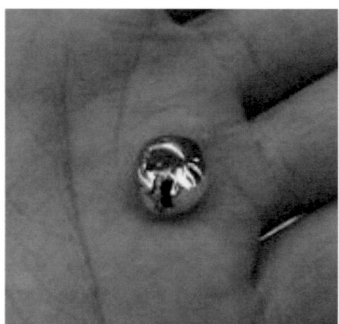

Figure 36: The removed crown.

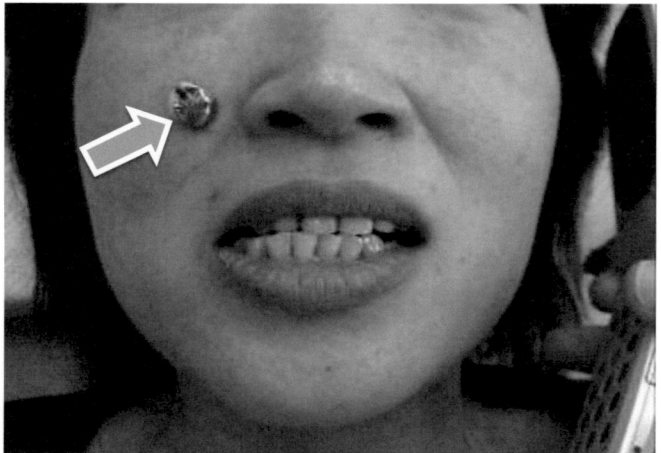

Figure 37: When the removal crown was placed on her cheek (arrow) and the active cell phone was brought close to her face, the involuntary movement recurred.

Discussion

The crown which was set on her right upper second molar might have been collecting harmful electromagnetic waves. The reason why the electromagnetic waves emitted by a cell phone can induce involuntary movement is not clarified yet. However, the electromagnetic waves seem to impede cranial nerve function, but further study is needed. The method for finding suspicious material using the Bi-Digital O-Ring Test is as follows: First, an active cell phone is placed near a subject. Second, a third person (nurse, hygienist etc.) touches the suspicious material with an electricity conducting prove while an O-ring is made with the other hand. Third, the doctor attempts to split the O-ring. If O-ring is easily spilit, the material may be collecting harmful electromagnetic waves (Figure 38).

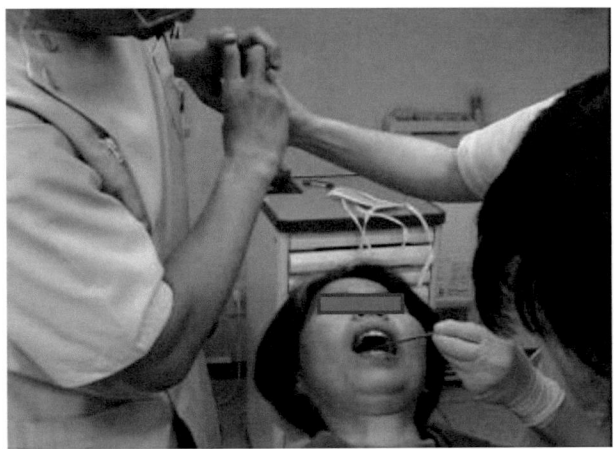

Figure 38: The third person (nurse, hygienist etc.) touches the suspicious material with an electricity conducting proves while an O-ring is made with the other hand. The doctor attempts to split O-ring. An active cell phone is placed on the dental desk, near the subject.

With regard to the relationship between brain tumors and electromagnetic waves emitted by cell phones, the Interphone Study Group had concluded that there was no increase in the risk of developing glioma or meningioma with the use of mobile phones. The authors also found that there were suggestions of an increased risk of glioma at the highest exposure levels; however, bias and error prevent a causal interpretation. Thus, the possible effects of long-term heavy use of mobile phones require further investigation [24]. Moreover, the WHO/International Agency for

Research on Cancer (IARC) has classified radiofrequency electromagnetic fields as Group 2B (agents that are possibly carcinogenic to humans), based on an increased risk for glioma, a malignant type of brain cancer associated with wireless phone use, in 2011 [25]. Other reports, similarly, do not support an association between the use of cell phones and the development of brain or salivary gland tumors, leukemia, or other cancers [26-28]. However, these reports did not sufficiently evaluate the risks among long-term heavy cell phone users over long induction periods [26]. Accordingly, further studies are required to account for longer exposure periods, particularly with respect to slow-growing intracranial tumors [27].

## Case 7: Difficulty of head movement

Subject, Methods, and Results

The subject was a woman in her 60's. Her right upper gums were swollen and festering because of an infected second premolar root (Figure 39). She could turn her head to the right sufficiently (Figure 40), but not to the left due to tension in her neck (Figure 41).

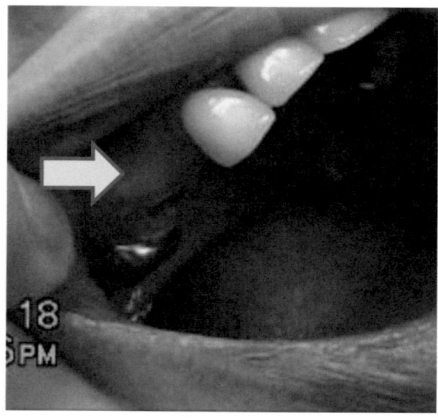

Figure 39: Her right upper gums were swollen and festering (arrow).

When I brought antibiotics, which were known to be effective on the pathogen, close to her right cheek, she could turn her head to the left more easily (Figure 42). As a result, I extracted the infected tooth root and the ailment was cured.

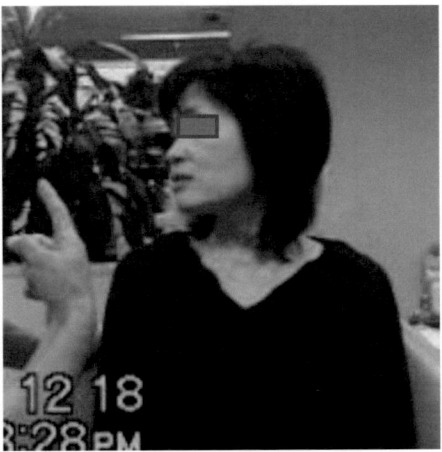

Figure 40: She could turn her head right easily.

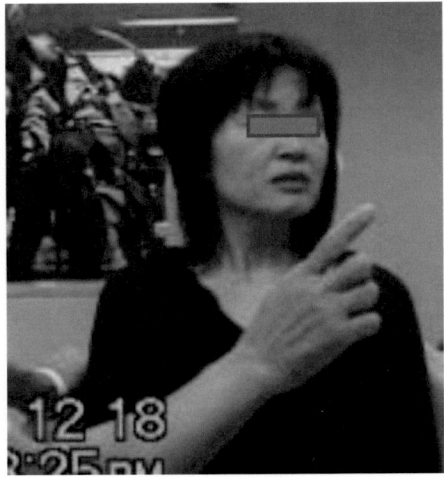

Figure 41: She could not turn her head left easily due to tension in her neck.

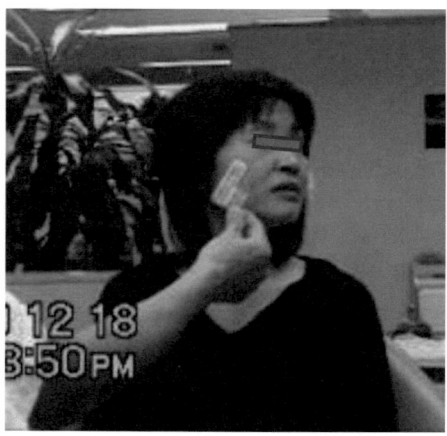

Figure 42: When antibiotics were brought close to her right cheek, she could turn her head to the left easily

Discussion

The bacteria in the patient's infected area might have been having an effect on her neck, and the antibiotics might have been effective on the bacterial infection. Her head movement disorder might have been due to something like a focal infection since the antibiotics were effective on her neck. This case shows that even when substances, including medicines, are not absorbed by the body, they can have a marked effect. I advocate that this effect should be called the indirect effect. Cases 1 and 2 show the indirect effect of dental materials. Case 3 shows the indirect effect of medicine. So far, this effect has been labelled as a placebo effect because it is believed that medicine will never work unless it entire the body.

In order to watch the actual experiment described in this case, please visit the YouTube movie:
Neck pain and stiffness are improved by bringing antibiotics close to the body.
https://www.youtube.com/watch?v=IsOnh4vpOBM&feature=youtu.be
(last checked: 8 Jan 2015)

# Case 8: Effect of magnetic field on the body

Subject and Methods

This case is a clinical case of a friend of mine, a dentist, but it's very interesting, so I'll introduce it. The subject was a woman in her 50's. Her chief complaint was severe dizziness. She had an upper full denture. When she wore the full denture, she felt dizzy. When the denture was removed, her symptom improved. There are two magnetic objects (permanent static magnets) in her upper full denture to retain and stabilize the denture (Figure 43).

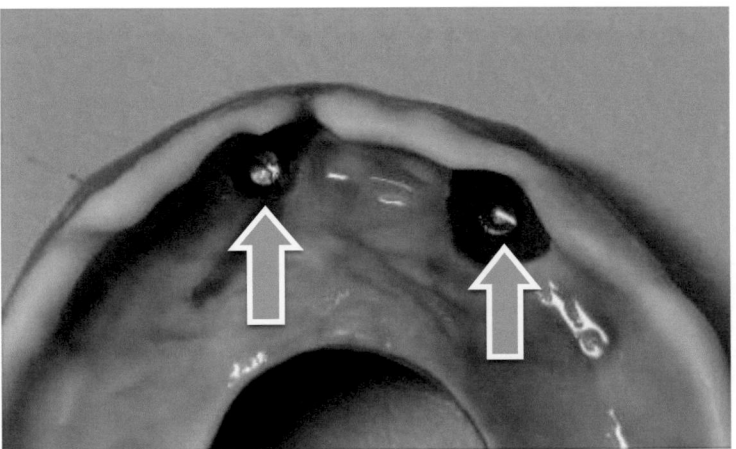

Figure 43: There are two magnetic objects (arrows) in her upper full denture to retain and stabilize the denture

In an X-ray image, there are two metal objects (arrows) which the magnetic materials attached to, on the teeth roots (Figure 44). The Dentist in charge thought that the magnetic objects were the cause of her symptoms by the Bi-Digital O-Ring Test [2, 3]. Therefore, he removed the magnetic objects (Figure 45).

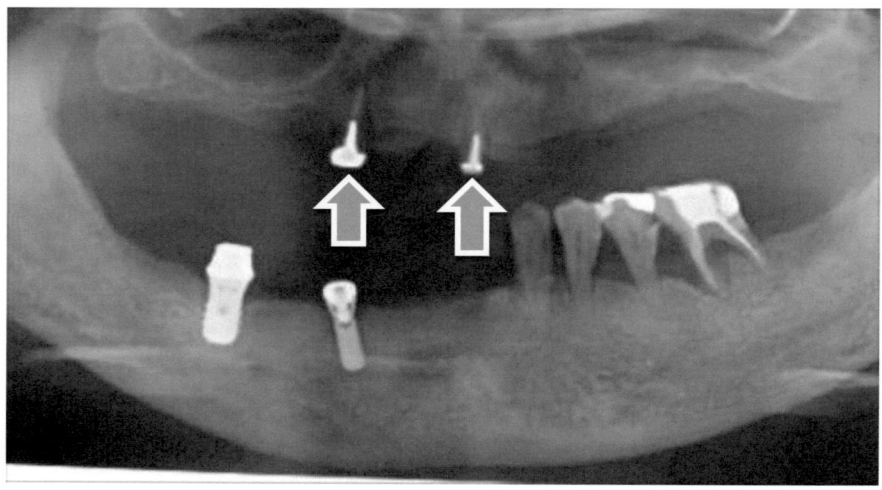

Figure 44: In an X-ray image, there are two metal objects (arrows) which the magnetic materials attached to, on the teeth roots.

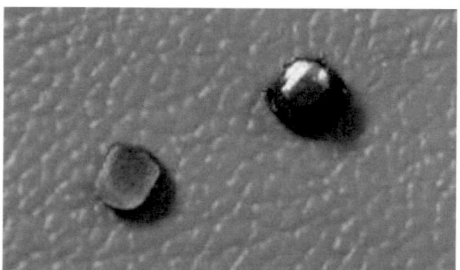

Figure 45: Removed magnetic objects (permanent static magnets).

Results

Her symptoms improved soon after removal of the magnetic objects from her upper full denture although the subject wore the full denture. In addition, when the removed magnetic objects were placed on her chest (arrow), her SLR and left hip joint mobility were decreased (Figure 46) and she felt tension.

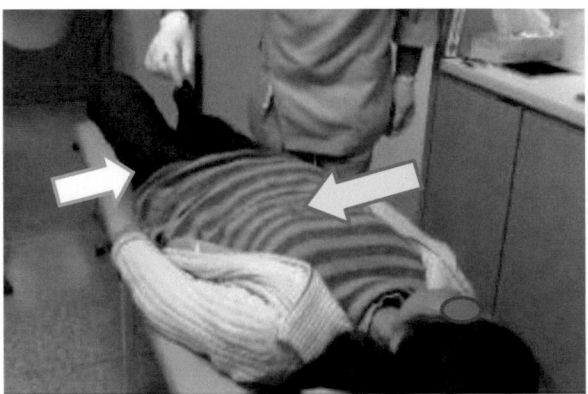

Figure 46: When removed magnetic objects (right arrow) were placed on the subject's chest, her right hip joint mobility was restricted due to tension (left arrow).

As soon as the magnetic objects were removed, her left hip joint movement and SLR returned to normal (Figure 47). Since this treatment, her symptoms have disappeared and have never reoccurred.

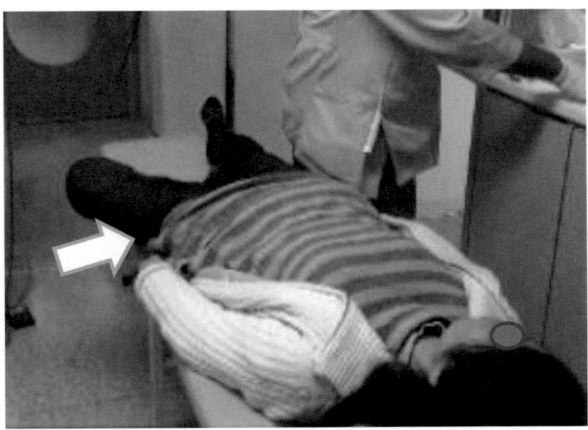

Figure 47: As soon as the magnetic objects were removed, the movement of her left hip joint became more flexible (arrow).

Discussion

The current case suggests that magnetic fields sometimes have an adverse effect on the body. Her symptoms, i.e. dizziness and joint mobility dysregulation might be caused by the harmful magnetic field. If the body is influenced by the magnetic field for a long time, like in this case, we should consider the effect of the magnetic field on the body. Magnet therapy exists and is classified as a pseudoscientific alternative medical practice. Magnet therapy is the application of the magnetic field of electromagnetic devices or permanent static magnets to the body for purported health benefits. Some believers recognize different effects based on the orientation of the magnet; under the laws of physics, magnetic poles are symmetrical [29]. However, the efficacy of it is debatable [30]. These results of this case suggest that magnetic therapy would certainly have a big influence on the body, but it's necessary to pay significant attention to any side effects.

## Case 9: Indirect and direct effect of a small denture on the whole body

Subject, Methods, and Results

The subject was a woman in her 40's. She had small back pain and stiffness of shoulders. When I performed the SLR test on both her legs, she felt a small pain, and tension (Figure 48). She also had small pain and tension when inner and outer rotation of her hip joint was performed.
Her upper right first molar was missing (Figure 49). I made a small denture to restore the position (Figure 50). When the little denture was placed on her chest, all joint movement that I checked has improved (Figure 51).

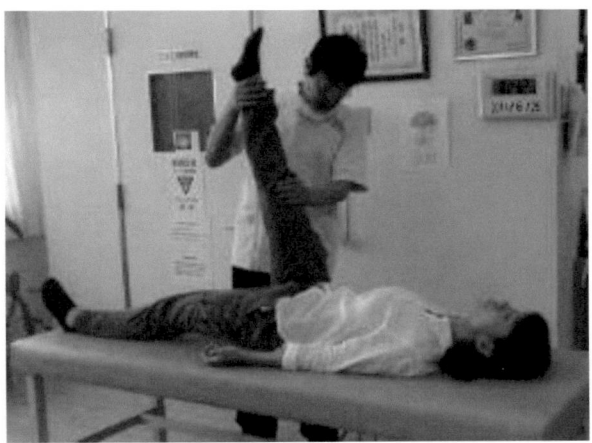

Figure 48: When the SLR test was performed on her right leg, she felt a small pain, and tension.

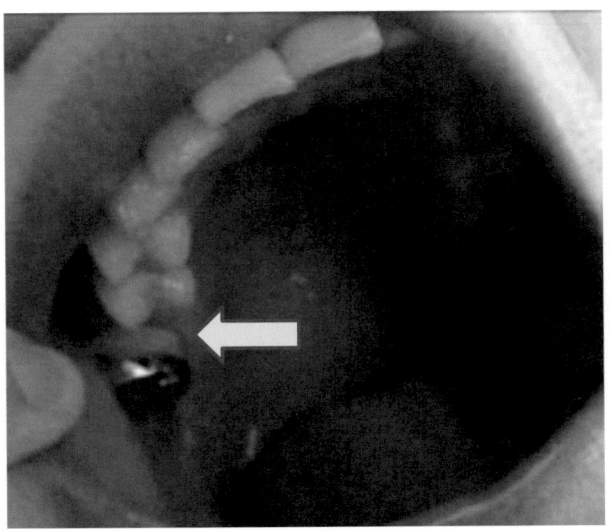

Figure 49: Her upper right first molar was missing (arrow).

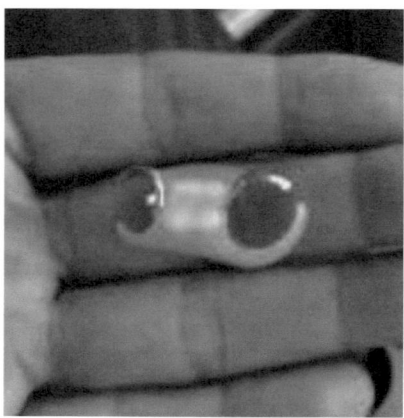

Figure 50: A little denture which would fill her missing position.

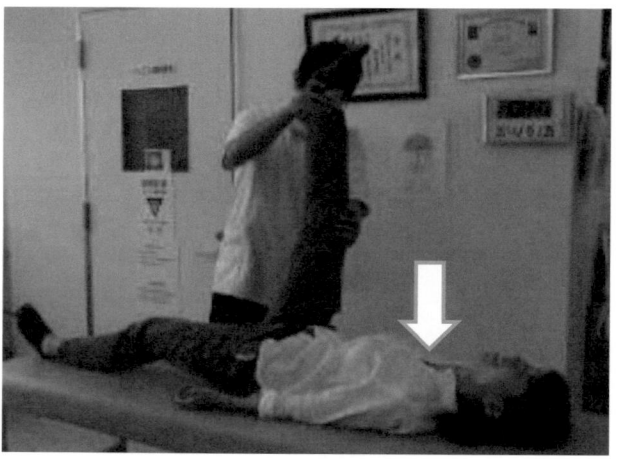

Figure 51: When the little denture was placed on her chest (arrow), all joint movement that I checked improved.

When she bent forward without her denture, the distance between her finger tips and the floor (FFD) was about 10cm (Figure 52). When the denture was placed near her feet, she was able to touch the floor with her fingertips (Figure53).

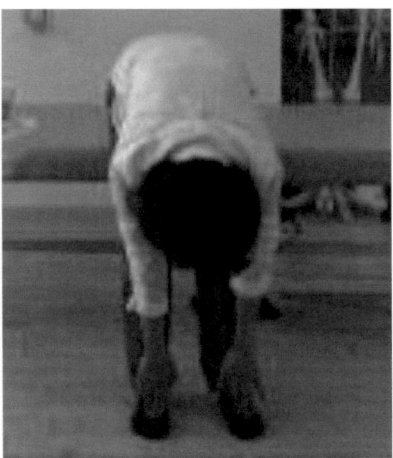

Figure 52: When she bent forward without her denture, the distance between her finger tips and the floor (FFD) was about 10cm.

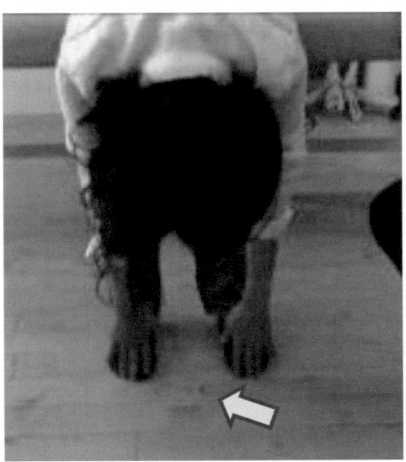

Figure 53: When the denture was placed near her feet (arrow), she was able to touch the floor with her fingertips.

When the denture was removed, the FFD returned. When I pushed her body from the side, she was very unstable (Figure 54). However, when the denture was placed near her feet, she became very stable (Figure 55).

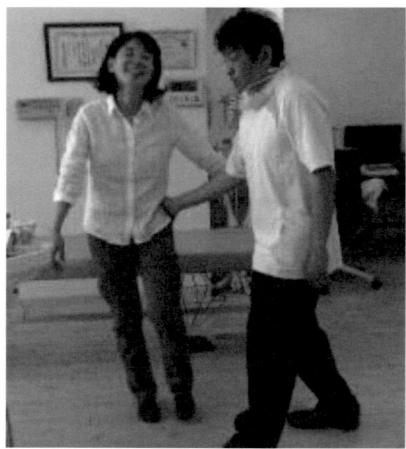

Figure 54: When her body was pushed, she was very unstable.

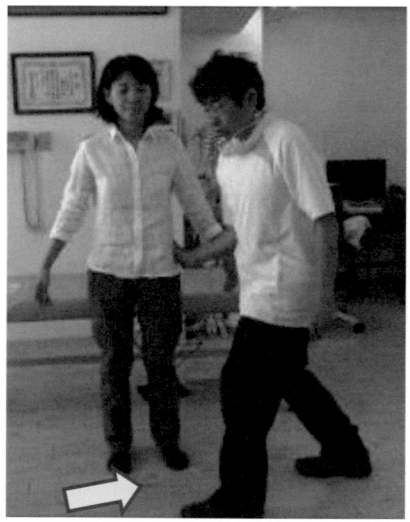

Figure 55: When the denture was placed near her feet (arrow), she became very stable.

When I removed the denture, she became unstable again. After the denture was placed in the missing position (Figure 56), all joint movement that I checked became more flexible than when the denture was near her body (Figure 57).

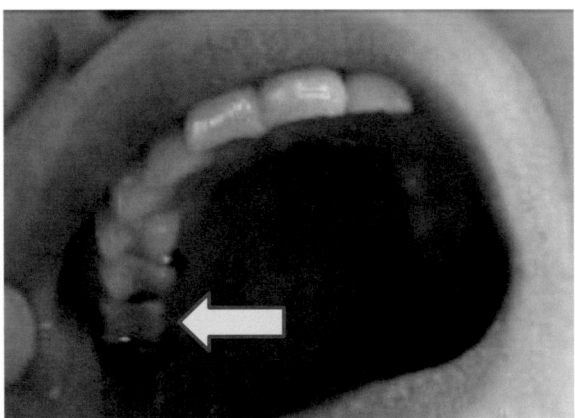

Figure 56: The denture was placed in her upper right molar position (arrow).

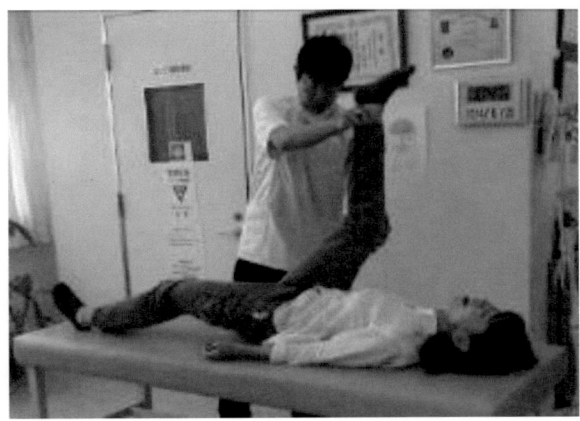

Figure 57: Her right leg rose more flexibly than when the denture was placed on her chest.

Her body became more stable than when the denture was placed near her body. Approximately 5 minutes after the denture was set in her mouth, her shoulders were looser and her body movement was easier.

Discussion

The current case also shows the direct and indirect effect of a small denture. The result of this case is similar to Case 1 and Case 2. However, this case clarifies that these effects may influence the body's stability. The method which I used to check the body's stability is very useful, i.e. when a researcher pushes a subject's body from sides, back, front, etc., we can observe how unsteady the subject's body is [31] [32]. Many diseases may be caused by spine malposture. Instability of the body may cause this spine malposture. Therefore, this pushing test may very important in evaluating evaluate body conditions before and after treatment.

In order to watch the actual experiment described in this case, please visit the You Tube movie:
Direct and indirect effects of a small denture on the body
https://www.youtube.com/watch?v=K10phUX9ur4
(last checked: 8 Apr. 2015)

## Case 10: Lumbago due a lumber vertebra herniated disc was treated by the indirect effect of medicine

Subject, Methods and Results

The subject was a woman in her 40's. She had a lumbago due to a lumber vertebra herniated disc (Figure 58). Her posture was leaned forward, and she could not keep her posture straight because of the lumbago (Figure 59). When the medicine, which was judged effective on her back by Bi-Digital O-Ring test [2][3], was placed on her back, she could straighten it (Figure 60)

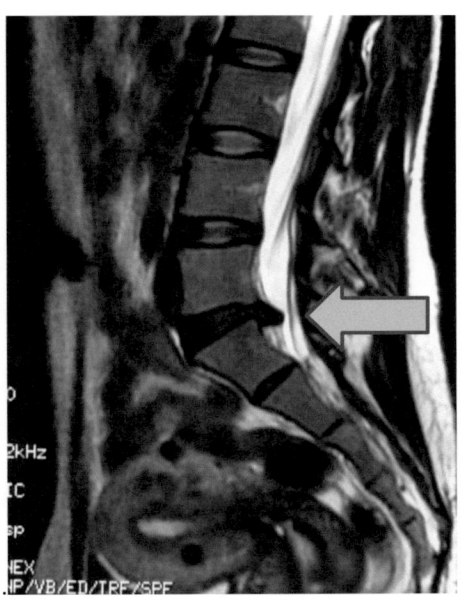

Figure 58: The subject had lumbago due to a lumber vertebra herniated disc in MRI (arrow).

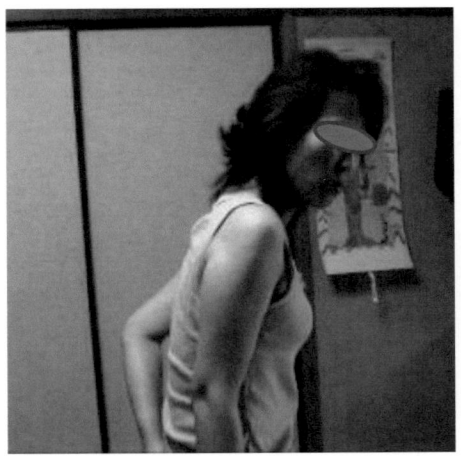

Figure 59: Her posture was leaned forward and she could not keep her posture straight because of the lumbago

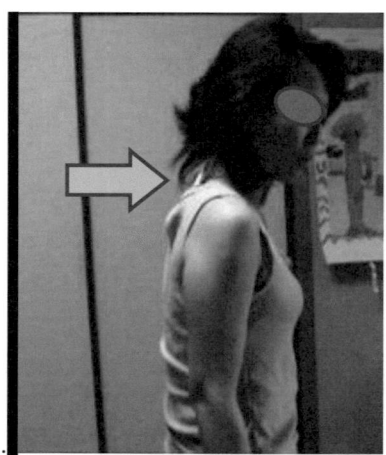

Figure 60: When the medicine which was judged effective on her back by Bi-Digital O-Ring test was placed on her back (arrow), she could straighten it.

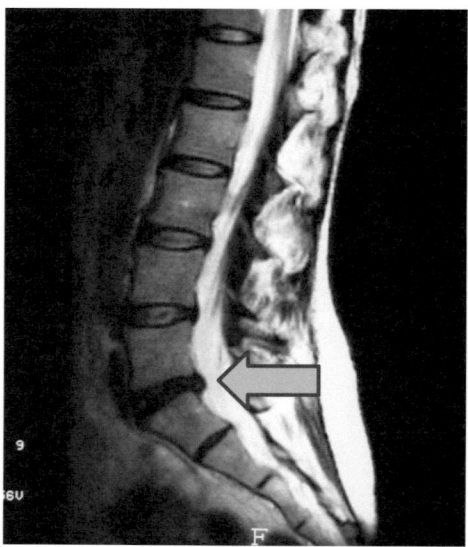

Figure 61: The lumber vertebra herniated disc improved (arrow) in MRI after treatment.

I suggested her to patch this medicine to reduce the pain of the lumbago when I conducted occlusal treatment. About 3 months after beginning the treatment, the lumbago was cured. The lumber vertebra herniated disc was improved in the MRI which was taken after that (Figure 61).

In order to watch the actual experiment described in this case, please visit the YouTube movie:
Lumbago was improved by the indirect effect of medicine
https://www.youtube.com/watch?v=dqZIizMDQ70
  (last checked: 16 Apr 2015)

Discussion

This case is also about the indirect effect of the medicine. There are some advantageous points in using the indirect effect. First it is very easy to apply because the medicine should be placed on the patient's body or affected area. Second, it is advantageous financially because the medicine is not ingested in the body. Third, it is easy to quit the treatment because the medicine is easy to remove. However, it is still unclear which is better, using the direct effect, indirect effect, or using both effects. I think if we have enough success with the indirect effect, we need not take medicine. However, we don't have enough success using the indirect effect, we should use the direct effect or both effects. In the current case, I achieved enough success using only the indirect effect. I suggested the patient patch the medicine on the affected area. However, if the patient does not see enough improvement, she would take the medicine. Such a method hasn't been established up until now, so it would seem it should be considered in a positive light from now on.

Overall discussion

There is a physical condition control method in which garlic is hung from the neck to prevent the flu and cold in Russia. I think this also anticipated the indirect effect of garlic (Figure 62). "Ring a Ring o' Roses" or "Ring Around the Rosie" is a nursery rhyme or folksong and playground singing game. One of the darker rhymes in the Mother Goose canon, "Ring Around the Rosy" refers to the bubonic plague, which ravaged Europe several times between the fourteenth and nineteenth centuries. Symptoms of the plague included a "rosy" red rash in the shape of a ring on the skin, hence the lyrics "ring around the rosy." Because of the popular belief that the disease was transmitted by foul odors, people carried pockets full of sweet herbs ("pocketful of posies") to repel the infection. This song may suggests the indirect effect of the posy (Table 1). It's called "FUKUYOU" to take medicine in Japan. "FUKU" means 'clothes' and "YOU" means 'using'. It may suggest that medicine should be patched to the body like clothes. Such a concept was ignored by modern Western medicine. If the body reacts by indirect effect, it has been recognized as the placebo effect.

Table 1

| Ring-a-ring-a-roses, A pocket full of posies; |
| Hush! hush! hush! hush! We're all tumbled down. |

*Ring A-Ring O' Roses – English Children's Song*

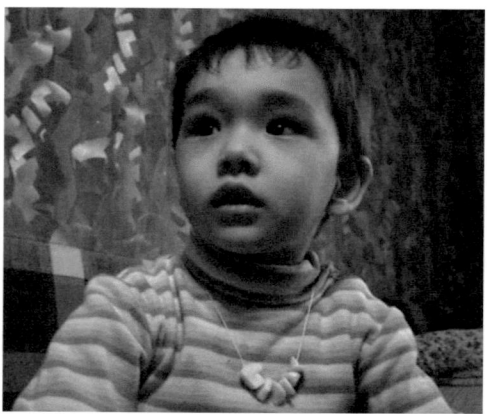

Figure 62: There is physical condition control method which garlic is hanged from a neck to prevent a flu and cold in Russia.
Cited from http://blogs.yahoo.co.jp/kat_perevod/9177086.html

My experiments have revealed that when the substances are simply in close proximity to the body, it indicates that medicine can influence a patient's condition in three ways: 1) the medicine can be absorbed by the cells, 2) it can have an effect when in close proximity to the body, and 3) it can cause a placebo effect. I am suggesting that the first mechanism be called the direct effect and the second be called the indirect effect of the medicine. Therefore, the outcome of taking any medicine will be the sum of the direct and indirect effects of the medicine on the patient. The indirect effect can have serious implications for the accuracy of the testing of new drugs. In the case of cohort studies, which are said to provide relatively high levels of evidence, subjects are divided into two groups. One group consists of those who take the medicine, and the other group consists of those who do not. The indirect effect could have unnoticed effects on such tests. For example, in the control group, some members may have medicine in their pockets. Despite the medicine being present in the pockets, real physical effects may be noticed on the individuals; such effects will not be classified as authentic by the investigators. These effects will be defined as placebo effects. When comparing effects, subjects should be classified into three groups: 1) those who took the medicine 2) those who had medicine in close proximity but did not take it, and 3) those from whom medicine is kept away and not taken. In randomized controlled trials (RCTs), a placebo is administered to some subjects, while the target medication is administered to others. The results are then compared. A placebo should have neither positive nor negative effects on subjects. However, if the placebo exerts a strong indirect effect on the body, the evaluation of the test medication could then be inaccurate. In summary, drug effectiveness measurements based on EBM (Evidence Based Medicine) cannot be trusted because of this indirect effect, which has not been accounted for in EBM to date [22]. The mechanism underlying the indirect effect remains unclear, further research is required. One hypothesis is that the indirect effect is the result of the unique electromagnetic waves emitted by every substance, including medicine. I believe that the mechanism which is causing the indirect effects on the subject is something like electromagnetic waves. That is, it can be blocked by aluminum foil, such as that used in the Case 1.

I have suggested that the electromagnetic waves emitted by cell phones and PCs may cause scoliosis, balance dysregulation, and joint mobility disorder [4] [20] [23]. I reported that the incidence of such issues decreased when aluminum foil was placed between an electromagnetic wave-emitting electronic device and the subject in Case 1 and other papers [4] [21] [23]. If there are severe side effects, the indirect effect could be much more effective than the direct effect. For example, medicine could be placed in the patient's pocket. The patient would receive the benefits of the indirect effect of the medicine without the side effects of the direct effect. In such a case, the efficacy of EBM for estimating the therapeutic value of medicine may be debatable. In another case, the placebo used by the control group may have noticeable indirect effects on the body. Moreover, in such a case, the results of past randomized controlled trials and cohort or case–control studies may be inaccurate. Even if the indirect effect has unwanted side effects, they can be quickly stopped by removing the medicine. This report has presented various cases that clearly show the indirect effects of dental materials and medicine. I hope to collect further evidence in the future in order to show that these results are wide-spread and quantifiable.

As the use of electronic devices continues to increase, EHS is sure to become a bigger issue [15-18]. In addition to the symptoms commonly associated with EHS (headaches, fatigue, tinnitus, dizziness, memory loss, irregular heartbeat, skin trouble, involuntary body movement and balance dysregulation), I have indicated that joint mobility disorder can be caused by EHS [4]. The best way to improve EHS symptoms seems to be avoidance of electromagnetic waves. I have also illustrated, one method for reducing exposure to electromagnetic waves involved is the removal and replacement of dental materials which attract and/or collect such waves [4][23]. Furthermore, this case shows how the Bi-Digital O-ring Test [2][3] can be a useful diagnostic tool for identifying materials which attract or collect electromagnetic waves, and how the same test can also be used to select the proper dental alloy for neutralizing harmful electromagnetic waves [4][21][23]. There are many aspects of these results for which the mechanism remains unclear. However, this approach has the potential to significantly improve the lives of some EHS patients.

# Conclusion

Information technology is developing dramatically all over the world. The number of cell phone and personal computer users has increased considerably in recent years; particularly in developed countries. These devices have facilitated communication on a global scale. However, there have been a number of reports of health problems related to the electromagnetic waves emitted by such electronic devices. Long lists of both general and severe symptoms, including headaches, fatigue, tinnitus, dizziness, memory loss, irregular heartbeat, and whole-body skin lesions, have been reported. These are reportedly associated with the condition known as electromagnetic hypersensitivity (EHS). There are not many papers which report the influences of electromagnetic waves on the whole body in dentistry. However, dental materials may act as antennas collecting harmful electromagnetic waves [4, 20, 23]. Moreover, dental materials may emit electromagnetic waves which effect the whole body or sometimes neutralize the harmful electromagnetic waves [20,21]. So far, these conditions have been ignored in dental research. However, from now on, these conditions should be given an attention because circumstances of electromagnetic waves become stronger. On the other hand, modern Western medicine has been ignoring the indirect effect. The techniques of evidence-based medicine (EBM) are being frequently used recently. Many scientists believe that EBM is the best method to evaluate the efficacy of medicine or medical treatment. The generally accepted theory of EBM is that if a medicine is not absorbed by the body, it will have no effect. Therefore, EBM has ignored the indirect effect, so the efficacy of EBM for estimating the therapeutic value of medicines may be debatable. Therefore, a more accurate evaluation method should be devised [22].

## References

[1] You Tube movie: Knee pain is reduced after a single treatment which only took several seconds
https://www.youtube.com/watch?v=QhVMvFrqa2c&feature=youtu.be
(last checked: 3/23/2015)

[2] OMURA YOSHIAKI, "Bi-digital O-ring test for imaging and diagnosis of internal organs of a patient", published 1993-02-23, issued 1993-02-23. US patent 5188107 http://academic.reed.edu/economics/parker/f11/354/pat/o-ring.pdf
(last checked: 2/16 /2015)

[3] http://bdort.org/ (last checked: 2/16/2015)

[4] Fujii, Y. (2015) Dental treatment for Dizziness and Joint mobility Disorder caused by Harmful Electromagnetic Waves. OJAPr, 3, 1-7.
DOI:10.4236/ojapr.2015.31001.
http://www.scirp.org/journal/PaperInformation.aspx?PaperID=54004
(last checked 4/30/2015)

[5] Geser, H. (2004) Towards a Sociological Theory of the Mobile Phone, Release 3.0, University of Zurich, (http://socio.ch/mobile/t_geser1.htm/).

[6] Van Dijk, J. and Hacker, K. (2003) The Digital Divide as a Complex and Dynamic Phenomenon, The Information Society, 19, 315-326.

[7] http://www.holistic-dentistry.net/blog/2013/07/entry_242/
(last accessed, 5/2/2014).

[8] Aalto, S., Haarala, C., Brück, A., Sipilä, H., Hämäläinen, H. and Rinne, JO (2006) Mobile Phone Affects Cerebral Blood Flow in Humans. J Cereb Blood Flow Metab, 26, 885-900.

[9] Feychting, M., Jonsson, F., Pedersen, N.L. and Ahlbom, A. (2003) Occupational Magnetic Field Exposure and Neurodegenerative Disease. Epidemiology, 14, 413-419.

[10] Håkansson, N., Gustavsson, P., Johansen, C. and Floderus, B. (2003) Neurodegenerative Diseases in Welders and Other Workers Exposed to High Levels of Magnetic Fields. Epidemiology, 14, 420-426.

[11] Ahlbom, A. (2001) Neurodegenerative Diseases, Suicide and Depressive Symptoms in Relation to EMF. Bioelectromagnetics, Suppl 5, 132-143.

[12] Linet, M.S., Hatch, E.E., Kleinerman, R.A., Robison, L.L., Kaune, W.T., Friedman, D.R., Severson, R.K., Haines, C.M., Hartsock, C.T., Niwa, S., Wacholder, S. and Tarone, R.E. (1997) Residential Exposure to Magnetic Fields and Acute Lymphoblastic Leukemia in Children. N Engl J Med, 337, 1-7.

[13] Röösli, M., Moser, M., Baldinini, Y., Meier, M. and Braun-Fahrländer, C. (2007) Symptoms of ill health ascribed to electromagnetic field exposure--a questionnaire survey. Int J Hyg Environ Health, 207, 141-150.

[14] Edelstyn, N. and Oldershaw, A. (2002) The acute effects of exposure to the electromagnetic field emitted by mobile phones on human attention. Neuroreport, 13, 119-121.

[15] Rea, W., Pan, Y., Yenyves, E., Sujisawa, I., Suyama, H., Samadi, N. and Ross, G. (1991) Electromagnetic Field Sensitivity. J Bioelectricity, 10, 241-256.

[16] Rubin, G.J., Das Munshi, J. and Wessely, S. (2005) Electromagnetic Hypersensitivity: A Systematic Review of Provocation Studies. Psychosom Med, 67, 224-232.

[17] Rubin, G.J., Das Munshi, J. and Wessely, S. (2006) A Systematic Review of Treatments for Electromagnetic Hypersensitivity. Psychother Psychosom, 75, 12-18.

[18] Norbert, L. (2009) Electromagnetic Hypersensitivity. Advances in Electromagnetic Fields in Living Systems, 5, 167-197.

[19] Kimata, H. (2005) Microwave Radiation from Cellular Phones Increases Allergen-specific IgE Production. Allergy, 60, 838-839.

[20] Fujii, Y. (2012) Do dental implants cause scoliosis?: A case report. Personalized Medicine Universe, 1, 79-80.
DOI: 10.1016/j.pmu.2012.05.012
http://www.personalizedmedicineuniverse.com/article/S2186-4950%2812%2900017-X/abstract
(last checked 4/30/2015)

[21] Fujii, Y.(2014) Gold alloy dental inlay for preventing involuntary body movements caused by electromagnetic waves emitted by a cell phone.
OJAPr, 2,37-43.4236/ns.2015.74019
DOI:10.4236/ojapr.2014.24005
http://www.scirp.org/journal/PaperInformation.aspx?PaperID=52248
(last checked 4/30/2015)

[22] Fujii, Y. : Calling into question the efficacy of Evidence-based medicine : Is it always the best approach? Is that really the placebo effect? Natural Science 7, 135-140.
DOI: 10.4236/ns.2015.74019.
http://www.scirp.org/journal/PaperInformation.aspx?PaperID=55272
(last checked 4/30/2015)

[23]Fujii, Y.(2014) Sensation of Balance Dysregulation Caused/Aggravated by a Collection of Electromagnetic Waves in a Dental Implant. OJAPr, 2, 29-35. DOI: 10.4236/ojapr.2014.23004.
http://www.scirp.org/journal/PaperInformation.aspx?PaperID=49928
(last checked 4/30/2015)

[24] Interphone Study Group (2010) Brain Tumor Risk in Relation to Mobile Telephone Use: Results of the Interphone International Case-control Study. Int J Epidemiol, 39, 675-694.

[25]WHO (2011) IARC Classifies Radiofrequency Electromagnetic Fields as Possibly Carcinogenic to Humans
http://www.iarc.fr/en/media-center/pr/2011/pdfs/pr208_E.pdf
(last checked 5/2/2014).

[26]Johansen, C., Boice, J.D. Jr, McLaughlin, J.K. and Olsen, J.H. (2001) Cellular Telephones and Cancer—a Nationwide Cohort Study in Denmark. J Natl Cancer Inst, 93, 203-207.

[27] Inskip, P.D., Tarone, R.E., Hatch, E.E., Wilcosky, T.C., Shapiro, W.R., Selker, R.G., Fine, H. A., Black, P.M., Loeffler, J.S. and Linet, M.S. (2001) Cellular-telephone use and brain tumors. N Engl J Med, 344, 79-86.

[28] Muscat, J.E., Malkin, M.G., Thompson, S., Shore, R.E., Stellman,S.D., McRee, D., Neugut, A.I. and Wynder, E.L. (2000) Handheld Cellular Telephone Use and Risk of Brain Cancer. JAMA, 284, 3001-3007.

[29] Rawls, Walter C.; Davis, Albert Belisle (1996). Magnetism and Its Effects on the Living System. Acres U.S.A. ISBN 0-911311-14-9.

[30] Magnet therapies 'have no effect'". *BBC*. 2006-01-06. Retrieved 2009-08-18.http://news.bbc.co.uk/2/hi/health/4582282.stm (last checked: 4/2/2015).

[31] https://www.youtube.com/watch?v=s35pViZvk-Q (last checked: 5/1/2015)

[32] https://www.youtube.com/watch?v=QHotr2lkbUY (last checked: 5/1/2015)

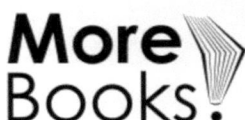

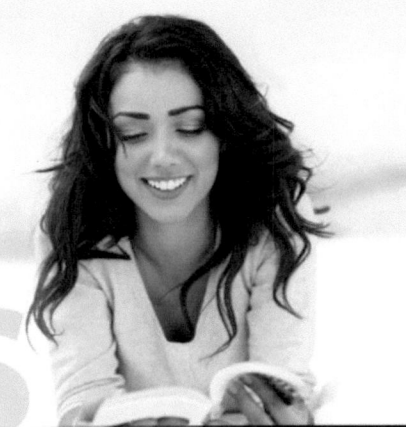

# I want morebooks!

Buy your books fast and straightforward online - at one of world's fastest growing online book stores! Environmentally sound due to Print-on-Demand technologies.

Buy your books online at
## www.morebooks.shop

Kaufen Sie Ihre Bücher schnell und unkompliziert online – auf einer der am schnellsten wachsenden Buchhandelsplattformen weltweit! Dank Print-On-Demand umwelt- und ressourcenschonend produziert.

Bücher schneller online kaufen
## www.morebooks.shop

info@omniscriptum.com
www.omniscriptum.com

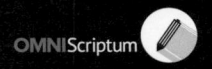

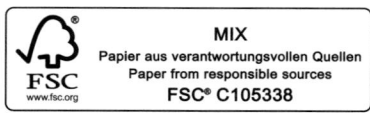

Printed by Books on Demand GmbH, Norderstedt / Germany